Hi

What ~~ ~erore, During And After

Rupert C. Robertson III

Copyright © 2015 - Rupert C. Robertson III

*

All rights reserved. No part of this book may be reproduced in any form or by any electronic or mechanical means including all information storage and retrieval systems without permission in writing from the author, except by a reviewer, who may quote passages in a review.

* * *

Table of Contents

Introduction

Initial Surprises

Pre-surgery

The surgery and hospital stay

The ride home

Getting home and setting up the house

The *list

Home therapy and recovery times

In The Future

Footnote

Introduction

When I first knew that I needed a hip replacement, I went to the internet to try to find what I could expect as far as the surgery itself, the amount of pain to expect, recovery times, quality of life after the surgery, possible side effects, etc. Much to my surprise, there just isn't much out there to tell you what to expect. The purpose of this article is to share my experiences of having a hip replaced and to give a little insight on what you might run into.

This is not my first experience with hip replacement. I first had my right hip done with a Burmingham Hip resurfacing procedure. (That's another paper.) About five years after I had my right hip done, I started experiencing severe pain in the area of my left hip. I let it progress to the point where I could only walk with the assistance of a cane and only barely then.

Since I was a veteran, the first place that I went was to the VA in my area. They did the usual examinations and I was told that my hip joint was "bone on bone" and that I needed a hip replacement. At the time, I was 67. I asked if they would do the surgery and my appointed VA doctor told me that I was too fat and needed to lose thirty pounds before they would even consider doing anything. I asked the doctor how I was supposed to exercise when I couldn't even walk and was told, in so many words, that it was my problem and to come back when I had lost the weight.

By the time I turned 68, the pain was to the point that my attitude was so bad that my wife was threatening to kill me if I didn't get something done. I started researching doctors in the private sector. Through the recommendation of several people, including an old friend that was a retired orthosurgeon, and a lot of on-line studying of different facilities, I finally decided on the Arkansas Surgical Hospital and Dr. William Hefley, Jr. as the group that I wanted to do my hip.

Initial Surprises

When I initially called Dr. Hefley's office to set up the actual procedure, I found out that it wasn't quite that simple. I was told that I would need clearance from a dentist before I could set up the surgery. Why? It turns out that having a dentist give you a clean bill of health lessens your chance of infection after the surgery.

After having a tooth pulled, a round of antibiotics and then an additional dental appointment for further exams and procedures, I finally got clearance from my dentist. Just so you know, this release is only good for six months and then you will have to start all over.

You also have to quit smoking 6 weeks prior to the surgery and they take you off most vitamins, aspirin, most pain medications and a few other things 2 weeks prior to the surgery. You just thought that you hurt before. The pain was so bad that I actually chipped a tooth during the night from gritting my teeth.

Pre-surgery

About a week before the surgery, I was given appointments for a final physical, to go to a class on the procedure where everything would be explained and to meet with the surgical staff other than my primary surgeon. I met with the internist, the anesthesiologist, blood work people, the surgeon's nurse and anyone else that they wanted me to meet. This is not a bad thing. These are the folks that will be looking out for you. Be nice to them.

The doctor told me that he uses a procedure that is "minimally invasive". I laughed and asked what was minimal about it. He patiently explained that they didn't cut the muscle when they went in, which allowed for a quicker recovery and faster mobility. He went on to say that a physical therapist would not be necessary and that all that would be needed was walking and exercise to recover fully.

It is my personal belief that you stand a better chance of a good procedure if you feel like you have made the best possible choices for your care and are mentally satisfied with those choices. The group that I met with made me feel totally at ease with everything they talked about and I left feeling totally confident in my choice.

The surgery and hospital stay

The evening before surgery, I had to prep myself with special wipes. It was pretty inclusive of the entire body and the following morning, before I left the hotel and checked in, the entire procedure was repeated. Doing this reduces any risk of infection around the surgical site and I was meticulous in following directions.

The day finally arrives for the surgery. I'm told to report at 6:00 am. Yup, six o'clock in the morning. Thank goodness we had the foresight to spend the night at a close-by hotel and didn't try to drive down that morning. If you live more than a few miles from your hospital, I would advise that you do the same. Talk to your doctor to see if they have a relationship or an agreement with a particular hotel. Often, there will be major discounts offered.

On arrival, I checked in at the proper place and was sent to pre-op. I was given the starting course of anesthesia and was made comfortable for the remaining time until the procedure was to start. My wife was allowed back in pre-op with me until time to go. When the time came, I remember being wheeled into the operating arena and not a whole lot more. There were bits and pieces that came back, but nothing painful or worrisome. The next thing I knew, I was waking up in recovery. After a short stay, it was back to my room.

My legs were strapped to a rigid foam triangle looking thingy so that I couldn't move them and so that the hip was held in a fixed position. It was not comfortable and I gripped about it. Every time I needed to do something, it had to be removed so that I could get up. I was kept in this torture device for around 36 hours. It caused the heels on my feet to hurt due to the pressure and the angle of the bed. They brought me soft foam booties to relieve the pressure and ease the pain.

My room was actually a suite and my wife had a pull out bed of her own so that she could stay with me. She had her own television and they even brought her heated blankets when she got chilled.

The physical therapist came in that afternoon with the idea of getting me up and going. It wasn't a long walk, but I did go out into the hall and back. It wasn't fun and it did hurt. I was also nauseous from the effects of the anesthesia and that didn't help. Then it was back to bed and get strapped back into the torture device.

Between therapy sessions, they put me on a leg squeezing device called an Activecare SFT calf pump, which is supposed to be worn for 22 hours a day for 14 days. This thing will drive you nuts but it helps prevent blood clots. It is noisy and has tubes that get in the way when you try to go anywhere. You will get used to it but you will never like it.

Let me insert a heads-up here. I was brought a plastic device with a bubble in it and was given a schedule to blow in it every so often. The person that brought it said that it was to make sure my lungs were functioning okay. I didn't think that I needed it and put it aside. What they failed to mention was that using it helped to clear the effects of the anesthesia out of the system. Use it and it will reduce any side effects, such as nausea, that you feel.

The next morning, about 24 hours after surgery, therapy began in earnest. The catheter was removed and I was picked up in a wheelchair and taken to the therapy suite. Once there, I was given a walker to pull up on and I was put through a variety of motion exercises and was asked about pain associated with different movements, etc. Rules were laid down about certain motions and movements that I should <u>not</u> do. I wasn't allowed to cross my legs, even lying down, no bending at the waist that went over 90 degrees, no pivoting. Basically, don't do anything that would put a backward or outward stress on the hip joint. Reason: it can pop out of joint if too much stress is exerted before the muscles are strong enough to hold it in place. See the *list.

I was then told to go up and down a small set of stairs and to walk around the room using the walker and was then taken back to my room. Pain levels at this point were non-existent because the doctor wanted me to be comfortable. The epidural was left in at a reduced level so that I could function but be pain free. That afternoon, the therapist came to the room with a walker and we walked to the therapy session where we went through the same basic routine of that morning. (Note: During all of this, I was getting up to go to the bathroom on my own and without supervision except for the first time. I even snuck in a very careful shower. My wife did keep an eye on me but didn't interfere.)

The following morning's session consisted mostly of laps around the hospital floor using a walker and that afternoon was mostly the same. They wanted to make sure that I could function on my own. By that time, I had asked to stop with the pain medication for reasons I will tell you about later. The next morning I was released from the hospital. I could have gone the afternoon before but my health insurance insisted that I stay the extra day. My release came about 65 hours after surgery.

The ride home

The ride home was rough. We live in the hills about 90 miles away from the hospital. The roads are crooked and bumpy the entire way. Needless to say, I was uncomfortable the entire trip. The pain was not severe but I did hurt. My wife is a great driver and she missed most of the pot holes but the constant jarring from side to side was constant. I wedged myself in as best as I could and tried to enjoy the scenery. Being comfortable was not an option.

Getting home and setting up the house

I was sent home with a supply of medications and the leg squeezing device. There was blood thinner, two types of pain medications (which I kept, just in case) and a stool softener. I added to those BCAAs Amino Acids. They are supposed to help muscle tissue redevelop, strengthen and tone quicker. I was also given a long *list of things not to do.

There are a few additional items that will be nice to have on hand once you get home.

Walker and/or crutches and cane (must have)
Potty extender (must have)
Body wipes or other means of keeping clean until you can shower
Gauze and tape
Alcohol and hydrogen peroxide

When you get into your house you are going to discover that the corridors, doors, halls, areas between furniture, etc. in your house have nothing that resembles the open space in your hospital room. Everything is narrower and more crooked. There is no such thing as a straight line between point A and point B. If you have pets; they will always lie in the area that you are trying to get through and insist on going with you everywhere while weaving between your legs as you try to walk.

You will (probably) also discover that the medication for pain causes constipation. After my experience the last time, I was off of the pain pills before I came home. (The last time, the stool softeners that they gave me didn't seem to work, so we bought a natural laxative (SennaGen) and when I finally got around to going (about 5 days later) I thought I was giving birth to a concrete bowling ball. It was the worse pain of anything associated with the surgery that I experienced.) I did take a pain pill whenever I did something stupid and caused a lot of pain, but I tried to minimize that as much as possible and only took a total of 4 pills during the entire recovery.

I'm lucky that my wife is not squeamish and was able to change the dressings every day for me. She cleaned it with alcohol and hydrogen peroxide and taped gauze over the wound. There was very little to no drainage and it was a fairly easy and quick procedure. She also applied antibiotic crème and a little vitamin E oil to reduce scarring. It must have worked, because you can barely make out the scar at all now a year later.

The *list

(As given to me.)

1. Avoid hip adduction (movement away from the body's center line) and external rotation.
2. Do not bend over to tie your shoes during the first 3 months.
3. You should not sit for more than 1 hour without standing and stretching as you have been taught.
4. When sitting, sit with your knees comfortably apart.
5. For 3 months, do not sit in very low chairs. You will find that this will require an excessive amount of hip flexion and, in the early months, may make your hip sore.
6. Do not lie on either side for the first 3 weeks following your surgery. You may, however, place 2 pillows between your knees to turn over to the prone position frequently. Lying on the side places undue stress on the components and may cause the hip to be sore.
7. It is safe for most people to return to driving 6 weeks following their surgery. A good guide for

this is when you have good leg control and can move your extremities from the gas pedal to the brake without significant effort.

8. Resumption of sexual intercourse is usually comfortable 4 to 6 weeks following discharge from the hospital.

9. 6 weeks following your discharge you should start a new exercise which is called side-lying abduction (aligned with the body's center line). One lies on the un-operated hip side with the operated hip side up. When assuming this position, place 2 pillows between your knees. The exercise itself is simply straightening the operated leg (which should be in line with the body) and lifting it toward the ceiling. Your goal should be 15 repetitions per session, with 3 sessions per day. This may take several weeks before you are able to do this.

10. After 6 weeks, the use of a stationary bicycle is very beneficial to the overall rehabilitation of your new hip. I recommend that you try to ride a stationary bicycle at least twice a day with an objective if 15 minutes each session.

11. The use of an elevated commode seat is helpful during the first 6 weeks following your discharge from the hospital. This allows you to sit comfortably and be independent for bathroom use very early. As you hip mobility and muscle strength improves, the elevated commode seat can be discontinued if you wish.
12. You may have some aching discomfort in your hip and thigh for the first several weeks following your operation. This discomfort should resolve with rest and if it does not, then you should cease all exercises and rest for a day or two until the discomfort does resolve.
13. It is important to remember that prior to any major dental procedure, you should be treated with preventative antibiotics provide by your dentist, for a lifetime.
14. You may begin to shower 24 hours after your staples are removed. A shower is preferred over a bath for the first 6 weeks.
15. Finally, the key to your overall rehabilitation program is to seek comfort. You should continue to do your exercises daily and increase them as your comfort and mobility allow.

16. **Reasons you should notify my (your doctors) office**: If you develop a temperature of 101.0 or greater, if you develop pain in the back of the calf of your surgical leg, if you develop chest pain or any shortness of breath or if you have any excessive bleeding that soaks through your surgical dressing and does not stop with pressure application

Home therapy and recovery times

I guess that this is a good place to talk about pain. Before the surgery, the pain was intense. It felt like someone was running a white-hot knitting needle into the hip joint. It was constant unless I was totally still. Immediately after the surgery, there was still pain, but of a totally different nature. It felt like someone had bruised the whole hip area with a vengeance. The pain was dull compared to before the surgery and much easier to deal with. Like a bruise, the pain lessened by a few degrees each day. It was like night and day and the pain after surgery was nothing compared with before.

The first night at home was very uncomfortable. I had trouble sleeping anywhere but on a reclining sofa that we have that supported the back as well as the rest of the body. Trying to lie flat in bed without rolling over was impossible for me. This went on for about two weeks.

I set myself up in the living room on the reclining sofa and recovery began. Every trip to the bathroom was a pain because of the leg squeezer. I had to unplug it and drape it over the walker to get around. Therapy instructions from the doctor consisted of the following:
   1. Walk 3 – 4 times a day.

2. Do exercises 3 time a day at 15 repetitions per exercise. The exercises were to pump the ankle up and down, to press the knee flat against a surface while sitting on a flat surface and leaning back and butt squeezes to help tighten the muscles.

After a few days, I made myself go up and down the stairs to the bedroom below to get clothes and for the exercise. I began using a cane rather than the walker fairly often because it was easier to get around the house. (I actually quit using the walker after 6 days. It just got in the way.)

After about a week and a half, I got rid of the leg squeezer for good. That in itself was cause for celebration. I started doing laps around the local WalMart using a buggy as a walker until I (my body) got tired. Since it was my left hip that was replaced, I could also drive. It makes a difference on which side the surgery was done and whether you drive a standard or automatic. If you drive an automatic and your surgery was on your left side then you can return to driving faster than if your right side is the one affected. If your surgery was done on the right side, it means that you have to accelerate and break with the side that is impaired. I found that driving for an hour became uncomfortable because you are basically locked into one position for long periods of time

Something I need to mention. When you start getting around you may find that the other side of your body will develop aches and pains. (After my first hip was replaced, my other hip began hurting worse than the one where I had the surgery. I've was told that is was just my body adjusting back to a normal attitude.)

Two weeks after the surgery, I was pretty much back to full tilt and going strong. I did use a cane off and on but tried to get around without it. Around 2 ½ weeks after coming home, I went back to have the staples removed from the incision. This was a quick procedure (around 15 minutes) with little or no pain involved. The doctor said I was looking good and to keep up the good work (I was told that I was pushing too hard but it just felt so good to be able to get around.) I was officially given the okay to drive.

The site of the incision healed quickly and 3 weeks after coming home I could completely and fully shower. Happy days! I also was able to start sleeping in my bed.

My health insurance was set up so that I could use our local health club, so I went there to do my own advanced therapy. I downloaded from the internet a few suggestions and gave them to the trainer at the gym. She designed a program for me to use that not only worked on the hip but also worked on my upper body. After the first workout I was sore as all get-out, but not in places that had anything to do with the surgery.

A quick note about therapy: Do it. If you mess around and don't do your therapy, your recovery time will be much longer and your return to normal activities will take forever.

In The Future

Once you have recovered to the point to where you feel that you are back to normal, you may feel aches and pains in your back and hip area. I couldn't figure out why I was having these pains until my wife noticed the way that I was walking. She told me that I was walking the same way that I was before the surgery. I was still compensating for the hip pain that was no longer there and it was causing me problems.

She now drops back and walks behind me off and on and lets me know what I am doing. After years of pain, it is hard to change what the body remembers. I am having to consciously pay attention to my stride and how I walk now to avoid complications.

Buy new shoes! This is important. You have been walking in a way that has been dictated by your body in order to avoid pain. Your old shoes have been worn to follow that pattern of movement. If you wear them after surgery, they will skew your body to walk in the old pattern and will throw your body off, thus hindering a normal walking pattern.

Something that I recently discovered. Your body will develop a sort of memory of how you were walking when you were hurting. It seems to do this in order to take the least painful path toward getting around. Your body will retain this memory after surgery, so you will have to retrain yourself on how to walk upright instead of doing the zombie shuffle.

In future visits to dentists, etc. you will need to get antibiotics ahead of time in order to prevent infections that might settle in the hip. This includes getting your teeth cleaned. My next thing that I will do will be to see my doctor at the end of the year.

Footnote

Keep in mind, everyone's experiences will differ to some degree. This information is intended to give you a firsthand look at my familiarity with this procedure and what I went through.

As an update:

I am now walking without pain and my stamina has improved greatly. I am pain-free.

Printed in Great Britain
by Amazon